CW00474225

The Definitive Dinner Mediterranean Diet Cookbook for Beginners

A Simple Cookbook for Every Dinner Lovers, with Genuine and Healthy Recipes!

Hanna Briggs

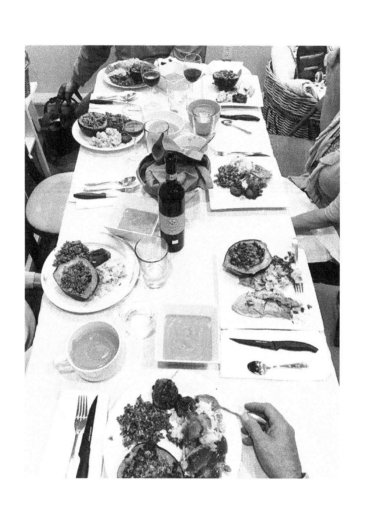

Table of contents

Introduction

Consuming the Mediterranean diet minimalizes the use of processed foods. It has been related to a reduced level of risk in developing numerous chronic diseases. It also enhances life expectancy. Several kinds of research have demonstrated many benefits in preventing cardiovascular disease, atrial fibrillation, breast cancer, and type 2 diabetes. Many pieces of evidence indicated a pattern that leads to low lipid, reduction in oxidative stress, platelet aggregation, and inflammation, and modification of growth factors and hormones involved in cancer.

Reduces Heart Diseases

According to research studies, the Mediterranean diet, which focuses on omega-3 ingredients and mono-saturated fats, reduces heart disease risk. It decreases the chances of cardiac death. The use of olive oil maintains the blood pressure levels. It is suitable for reducing hypertension. It also helps in combating the disease-promoting impacts of oxidation. This diet discourages the use of hydrogenated oils and saturated fats, which can cause heart disease.

Weight-loss

If you have been looking for diet plans for losing weight without feeling hungry, the Mediterranean diet can give you long term results. It is one of the best approaches. It is sustainable as it provides the most realistic approach to eat to feel full and energetic. This diet mostly consists of nutrient-dense food. It gives enough room for you to choose between low-carb and lower protein food. Olive oil consumed in this diet has antioxidants, natural vitamins, and some crucial fatty acids. It all improves your overall health. The Mediterranean diet focuses on natural foods, so there is very little room for junk and processed foods contributing to health-related issues and weight gain.

Most people trying the Mediterranean diet have gained positive results in cutting their weight. It is a useful option for someone looking forward to weight-loss as it provides the most unique and simple way to lose the overall calories without even changing your lifestyle that much. When you try to decrease calorie intake, losing weight is inevitable dramatically. But it will not benefit you. It will cause many health problems for you, including severe muscle loss. When you go for a Mediterranean diet, the body moves towards a sustainable model that burns calories slowly. So, it is crucial to practice the right approach and choose fat burning and more effective weight loss.

Prevents Cancer

The cornerstone of this diet is plant-based ingredients, especially vegetables and fruits. They help in preventing cancer. A plant-based diet provides antioxidants that help in protecting your DNA from damage and cell mutation. It also helps in lowering inflammation and delaying tumor growth. Various studies found that olive oil is a natural way to prevent cancer. It also decreases colon and bowel cancers. The plant-based diet balances blood sugar. It also sustains a healthy weight.

Prevents Diabetes

Numerous studies found that this healthy diet functions as an anti-inflammatory pattern, which helps fight the diseases related to chronic inflammation, Type 2 diabetes, and metabolic syndrome. It is considered very effective in preventing diabetes as it controls the insulin levels, which is a hormone to control the blood sugar levels and causes weight gain. Intake of a well-balanced diet consisting of fatty acids alongside some healthy carbohydrates and proteins is the best gift to your body. These foods help your body in burning fats more efficiently, which also provides energy. Due to the consumption of these kinds of foods, the insulin resistance level becomes non-existent, making it impossible to have high blood sugar.

Anti-aging

Choosing a Mediterranean diet without suffering from malnutrition is the most efficient and consistent anti-aging intervention. It undoubtedly expands lifespan, according to the research. The study found that the longevity biomarkers, i.e., body temperature and insulin level, and the DNA damage decreased significantly in humans by the Mediterranean diet. Other mechanisms also prove the claim made by researchers in explaining the anti-aging effects of adopting the Mediterranean diet, including reduced lipid peroxidation, high efficiency of oxidative repair, increased antioxidant defense system, and reduced mitochondrial generation rate.

Maintains Blood Sugar Level

The Mediterranean diet focuses on healthy carbs and whole grains. It has a lot of significant benefits. Consumption of whole-grain foods, like buckwheat, quinoa, and wheat berries instead of refined foods, helps you maintain blood sugar levels that ultimately gives you enough energy for the whole day.

Enhances Cognitive Health

The Mediterranean diet helps in preserving memory. It is one of the most useful steps for Alzheimer's treatment and dementia. Cognitive disorders occur when our brains do not get sufficient dopamine, which is a crucial chemical vital for mood regulation, thought processing, and body movements. Healthy fats like olive oil and nuts are good at fighting cognitive decline, mostly an age-related issue. They help counter some harmful impacts of the free radicals, inflammation, and toxins caused by having a low diet. The Mediterranean diet proves to be beneficial in decreasing

the risk of Alzheimer's to a great extent. Foods like yogurt help in having a healthy gut that improves mood, cognitive functioning, and memory.

Better Endurance Level

Mediterranean diet helps in fat loss and maintains muscle mass. It improves physical performance and enhances endurance levels. Research done on mice has shown positive results in these aspects. It also improves the health of our tissues in the long-term. The growth hormone also offers increased levels as a result of the Mediterranean diet. Which ultimately helps in improving metabolism and body composition.

Keeps You Agile

The nutrients from the Mediterranean diet reduces your risk of muscle weakness and frailty. It increases longevity. When your risk of heart disease reduces, it also reduces the risk of early death. It also strengthens your bones. Certain compounds found in olive oil help in preserving bone density. It helps increase the maturation and proliferation of the bone cells—dietary patterns of the Mediterranean diet help prevent osteoporosis.

Healthy Sleep Patterns

Our eating habits have a considerable impact on sleepiness and wakefulness. Some Mediterranean diet believers have reported an improved sleeping pattern as a result of changing their eating patterns. It has a considerable impact on your sleep because they regulate the circadian rhythm that determines our sleep patterns. If you have a regulated and balanced circadian rhythm, you will fall asleep quite quickly. You will also feel refreshed when you wake up. Another theory states that having the last meal will help you digest the food way before sleep. Digestion works best when you are upright.

Apart from focusing on plant-based eating, the Mediterranean diet philosophy emphasizes variety and moderation, living a life with perfect harmony with nature, valuing relationships in life, including sharing and enjoying meals, and having an entirely active lifestyle. The Mediterranean diet is at the crossroads. With the traditions and culture of three millennia, the Mediterranean diet lifestyle made its way to the medical world a long time ago. It has progressively recognized and became one of the successful and healthiest patterns that lead to a healthy lifestyle.

Besides metabolic, cardiovascular, cognitive, and many other benefits, this diet improves your life quality. Therefore, it is recommended today by many medical professionals worldwide. Efforts are being made in both non--Mediterranean and Mediterranean populations to make everyone benefit from the fantastic network of eating habits and patterns that began in old-time and which became a medical recommendation for a healthy lifestyle.

What to Eat and what to avoid

Fruits and vegetables: Mediterranean diet is one of the plant-based diet plans. Fresh fruits and vegetables contain a large number of vitamins, nutrients, fibers, minerals, and antioxidants

Fruits: Apple, berries, grapes, peaches, fig, grapefruit, dates, melon, oranges and pears.

Vegetables: Spinach, Brussels sprout, kale, tomatoes, kale, summer squash, onion, cauliflower, peppers, cucumbers, turnips, potatoes, sweet potatoes, and parsnips.

Seeds and nuts: Seeds and nuts are rich in monounsaturated fats and omega- 3 fatty acids.

 Seeds: pumpkin seeds, flax seeds, sesame seeds, and sunflower seeds. Nuts: Almond, hazelnuts, pistachios, cashews, and walnuts.

Whole grains: Whole grains are high in fibers and they are not processed so they do not contain unhealthy fats like trans-fats compare to processed ones.

Whole grains: Wheat, quinoa, rice, barley, oats, rye, and brown rice. You can also use bread and pasta which is made from whole grains.

Fish and seafood: Fish are the rich source of omega-3 fatty acids and proteins. Eating fish at least once a week is recommended here. The healthiest way to consume fish is to grill it. Grilling fish taste good and never need extra oil.

Fish and seafood: salmon, trout, clams, mackerel, sardines, tuna and shrimp.

Legumes: Legumes (beans) are a rich source of protein, vitamins, and fibers. Regular consumption of beans helps to reduce the risk of diabetes, cancer and heart disease.

Legumes: Kidney beans, peas, chickpeas, black beans, fava beans, lentils, and pinto beans.

Spices and herbs: Spices and herbs are used to add the taste to your meal.

Spices and herbs: mint, thyme, garlic, basil, cinnamon, nutmeg, rosemary, oregano and more.

Healthy fats: Olive oil is the main fat used in the Mediterranean diet. It helps to reduce the risk of inflammatory disorder, diabetes, cancer, and heart- related disease. It also helps to increase HDL (good cholesterol) levels and decrease LDL (bad cholesterol) levels into your body. It also helps to lose weight.

Fats: Olive oil, avocado oil, walnut oil, extra virgin olive oil, avocado, and olives.

Dairy: Moderate amounts of dairy products are allowed during the Mediterranean diet. The dairy product contains high amounts of fats.

Dairy: Greek yogurt, skim milk and cheese.

Food to avoid

Refined grains: Refined grains are not allowed in a Mediterranean diet. It raises your blood sugar level. Refined grains like white bread, white rice, and pasta.

Refined oils: Oils like vegetable oils, cottonseed oils, and soybean oils are completely avoided from the Mediterranean diet. It raises your LDL (bad cholesterol) level.

Added Sugar: Added sugar is not allowed in the Mediterranean diet. These types of artificial sugars are found in table sugar, soda, chocolate, ice cream, and candies. It raises your blood sugar level.

You should consume only natural sugars in the Mediterranean diet.

Processed foods: Generally Processed foods come in boxes. Its low-fat food should not be eaten during the diet. It contains a high amount of trans-fats. Mediterranean diet is all about to eat fresh and natural food.

Trans-fat and saturated fats: In this category of food contains butter and margarine.

Processed Meat: Mediterranean diet does not allow to use of processed meat such as bacon, hot dogs and sausage.

21 days meal plan with meal prep tips
Meal Preparation tips

Use extra-virgin olive oil instead of butter

Butter contains saturated fats. Saturated fats are not recommended during the Mediterranean diet. Instead of butter, you can use extra virgin olive oil. Olive oil is heart-healthy oil contains good fat like polyunsaturated and monounsaturated fats. You can also use olive oil over salad for dressing. Extra virgin olive oil is healthy fat recommended in the Mediterranean diet.

Add more avocados into your diet

Avocados contains healthy monounsaturated fats which is one of the good fats recommended in the Mediterranean diet.

Add whole grain and brown rice

 Mediterranean diet recommends brown rice and whole grains in the diet because grains are the best source of protein and they are rich in fibers. The bowl of oatmeal is one of the perfect breakfasts during the cold season.

Eat more legumes

Legumes are full of nutrients they are rich in fibers, high in proteins and low in fats. Legumes are also your budget-friendly food. It includes lentils, chickpeas, dried peas, and beans.

Consume plenty of fruits

Fruits are an essential part of the Mediterranean diet. Fruits are a good source of vitamins, fibers, and antioxidants. It is the best source of natural sugar and it is available easily. It helps to fulfill your sugar carving.

Don't overdo alcohol

Alcohol is part of the Mediterranean lifestyle. One of the misunderstandings is about alcohol is that you can drink lots of alcohol in the form of red wine. A moderate amount of alcohol is allowed while eating a meal.

Eat more fish

Fish is the best source of protein and omega-3 fatty acids. Specially eat fatty fish like mackerel, salmon, and sardines. One of the best ways to eat fish is to grill it. Grilled fish has great taste and never take extra oil for cooking.

Focus on the meal

While eating your meal you must concentrate on your meat. Always eat your meal slowly, give yourself 20 minutes to eat a meal. Stop eating your food in front of the television. You must focus and concentrate on your meal while eating.

Grocery list for each day

Now that you have begun taking steps towards integrating the Mediterranean diet into your lifestyle, the time has come to go shopping. Stocking your refrigerator and pantry with the right ingredients will go a long way to ensuring your success on this easy diet.

To make things easier for you and because I like to categorize, I've made a shopping list that will cover almost all your cooking needs:

Protein

Unsalted nuts

Fish and shellfish

Beans, peas, and lentils

Lean meats

Skinless chicken and poultry where possible

Poultry

Eggs

Dairy

All dairy should either be low-fat or fat-free.

Yogurt Sour cream

Almond milk Rice milk Hemp milk Soy milk

Cheese (try to find the reduced fat cheeses)

Spices

Salt Pepper Cinnamon Cumin

Chili powder Cayenne pepper Curry powder

 Honey Vinegar Garlic Ginger Herbs

Whole grains

Brown rice Quinoa

Whole grain bread Whole wheat pasta

Whole wheat flour, preferably stone milled Whole grain couscous

Vegetables

Fruit

Any fresh vegetables. Do try to incorporate a lot of dark leafy greens in your diet since they are full of antioxidants and other nutrients.

Frozen vegetables

Any fresh fruit that you enjoy. Aim to have seasonal fruits. This will help keep your budget cost-effective while you enjoy fresh produce.

Frozen fruit

Seeds Oatmeal Chickpeas Black beans

White beans

Low-sodium broth Other necessities

Dry red wine such as cabernet sauvignon Dark chocolate, roughly around the 70% mark Unsweetened cocoa

21 meal plan

Day 1

Breakfast: Italian Basil and Mushroom Omelet

Lunch: Provençal Vegetable Soup

Dinner: Steamed Italian Halibut with Green Grapes

Snacks: Tender Roasted Sweet Potatoes with Savory Tahini Sauce

Day 2

Breakfast: Mediterranean Fruit Oatmeal

Lunch: Grilled Chicken Salad with Fennel, Orange, and Raisins

Dinner: Hearty Root Veggie and Beef Stew

Snacks: Homemade Whole Wheat Pita Bread

Day 3

Breakfast: Smoked Salmon and Asparagus Omelet

Lunch: Simple Rosemary Shrimp Polenta

Dinner: Italian Chicken Stew with Potatoes, Bell Peppers and Tomatoes

Snacks: Crisp Spiced Cauliflower with Feta Cheese

Day 4

Breakfast: Mediterranean Muesli

Lunch: Tunisian Turnovers with Tuna, Egg and Tomato

Dinner: Eggplants with Tomato and Minced Lamb Stuffing

Snacks: Pumpkin Kibbeh

Day 5

Breakfast: Buckwheat Berry Crepes with Cottage Cheese

Lunch: Fish and Spinach Gratin

Dinner: Savory Roasted Sea Bass

Snacks: Oven Roasted Carrots with Olives and Cumin Yogurt Sauce

Day 6

Breakfast: No-Crust Broccoli and Cheese Quiche

Lunch: Calamari with Herb and Rice Stuffing

Dinner: Pork Roast with Zest Fig and Acorn Squash

Snacks: Bravas Potatoes with Roasted Tomato Sauce

Day 7

Breakfast: Banana-Strawberry Breakfast Smoothie

Lunch: Classic Niçoise Chicken

Dinner: Warm-Spiced Lamb Meatballs in Tomato Sauce

Snacks: Spring Peas and Beans with Zesty Thyme Yogurt Sauce

Day 8

Breakfast: Italian Basil and Mushroom Omelet

Lunch: Provençal Vegetable Soup

Dinner: Steamed Italian Halibut with Green Grapes

Snacks: Tender Roasted Sweet Potatoes with Savory Tahini Sauce

Day 9

Breakfast: Mediterranean Fruit Oatmeal

Lunch: Grilled Chicken Salad with Fennel, Orange, and Raisins

Dinner: Hearty Root Veggie and Beef Stew

Snacks: Homemade Whole Wheat Pita Bread

Day 10

Breakfast: Smoked Salmon and Asparagus Omelet

Lunch: Simple Rosemary Shrimp Polenta

Dinner: Italian Chicken Stew with Potatoes, Bell Peppers and Tomatoes

Snacks: Crisp Spiced Cauliflower with Feta Cheese

Day 11

Breakfast: Mediterranean Muesli

Lunch: Tunisian Turnovers with Tuna, Egg and Tomato

Dinner: Eggplants with Tomato and Minced Lamb Stuffing

Snacks: Pumpkin Kibbeh

Day 12

Breakfast: Buckwheat Berry Crepes with Cottage Cheese

Lunch: Fish and Spinach Gratin

Dinner: Savory Roasted Sea Bass

Snacks: Oven Roasted Carrots with Olives and Cumin Yogurt Sauce

Day 13

Breakfast: No-Crust Broccoli and Cheese Quiche

Lunch: Calamari with Herb and Rice Stuffing

Dinner: Pork Roast with Zest Fig and Acorn Squash

Snacks: Bravas Potatoes with Roasted Tomato Sauce

Day 14

Breakfast: Banana-Strawberry Breakfast Smoothie

Lunch: Classic Niçoise Chicken

Dinner: Warm-Spiced Lamb Meatballs in Tomato Sauce

Snacks: Spring Peas and Beans with Zesty Thyme Yogurt Sauce

Day 15

Breakfast: Italian Basil and Mushroom Omelet

Lunch: Provençal Vegetable Soup

Dinner: Steamed Italian Halibut with Green Grapes

Snacks: Tender Roasted Sweet Potatoes with Savory Tahini Sauce

Day 16

Breakfast: Mediterranean Fruit Oatmeal

Lunch: Grilled Chicken Salad with Fennel, Orange, and Raisins

Dinner: Hearty Root Veggie and Beef Stew

Snacks: Homemade Whole Wheat Pita Bread

Day 17

Breakfast: Smoked Salmon and Asparagus Omelet

Lunch: Simple Rosemary Shrimp Polenta

Dinner: Italian Chicken Stew with Potatoes, Bell Peppers and Tomatoes

Snacks: Crisp Spiced Cauliflower with Feta Cheese

Day 18

Breakfast: Mediterranean Muesli

Lunch: Tunisian Turnovers with Tuna, Egg and Tomato

Dinner: Eggplants with Tomato and Minced Lamb Stuffing

Snacks: Pumpkin Kibbeh

Day 19

Breakfast: Buckwheat Berry Crepes with Cottage Cheese

Lunch: Fish and Spinach Gratin

Dinner: Savory Roasted Sea Bass

Snacks: Oven Roasted Carrots with Olives and Cumin Yogurt Sauce

Day 20

Breakfast: No-Crust Broccoli and Cheese Quiche

Lunch: Calamari with Herb and Rice Stuffing

Dinner: Pork Roast with Zest Fig and Acorn Squash

Snacks: Bravas Potatoes with Roasted Tomato Sauce

Day 21

Breakfast: Banana-Strawberry Breakfast Smoothie

Lunch: Classic Niçoise Chicken

Dinner: Warm-Spiced Lamb Meatballs in Tomato Sauce

Snacks: Spring Peas and Beans with Zesty Thyme Yogurt Sauce

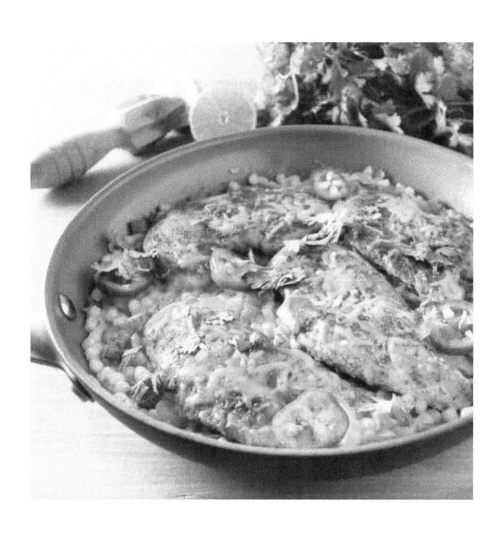

Greek Almond Rounds Shortbread

Servings: 20

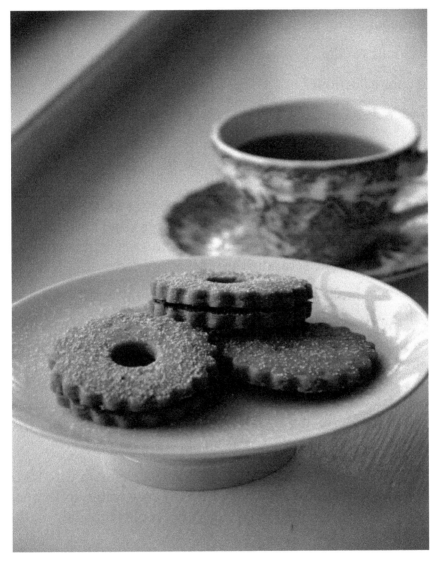

Ingredients

1/2 cups butter, softened

cup blanched almonds, lightly toasted and finely ground cup powdered sugar egg yolks

tablespoons brandy or orange juice

tablespoons rose flower water, (optional)

teaspoons vanilla

1/2 cups cake flour

Powdered sugar

Directions:

1.   Using an electric mixer, beat the butter on MEDIUM or HIGH speed for about 30 seconds in a large sized bowl. Add the 1 cup powdered sugar; beat until the mixture is light in color and fluffy, occasionally scraping the bowl as needed.

2.   Beat in the yolks, vanilla, and the brandy until combined.

3.   With a wooden spoon, stir in the flour and almonds until well incorporated. Cover and refrigerate for about 1 hour or until chilled and the dough is easy to handle.

4.   Preheat the oven to 325F.

5.   Place the cookie sheet into the preheated oven; bake for about 12-14 minutes or until the cookies are set.

6.   When the cookies are baked, transfer them on wire racks. While they are still warm, brush with the rose water, if desired. Sprinkle with more powdered sugar. Let cool completely on the wire racks.

Frozen Mediterranean Delight

Servings: 4

Ingredients

6 pitted dates, chopped

3 cups yogurt, plain, nonfat

2/3 cup pistachios, natural, unsalted, shelled

2 ounces bittersweet chocolate

1/2 cup sugar tablespoon ouzo

Directions:

1.   Line a fine meshed strainer with cheesecloth. Place the strainer over a bowl. Put the yogurt in the cheesecloth lines strainer; allow to drain for 2 hours.

2.   Put the sugar and half of the pistachios in a coffee grinder or a food processor, grind or process until powder.

3.   Roughly chop the remaining pistachios.

4.   Combine the drained yogurt, nuts, sugar-pistachio mixture, ouzo, and dates, mixing until well incorporated; place in the freezer. After 1 hour, remove from the freezer and mix well. Return to the freezer and freeze until firm.

5.   Divide into 4 servings. Garnish with chocolate shavings; serve

Mediterranean Scallops

Servings: 4

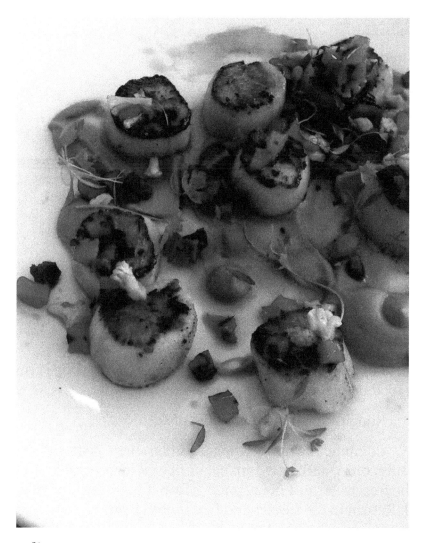

Ingredients:

8 to 12 ounces whole-wheat linguine

2 teaspoons garlic, minced

2 tablespoons shallots, minced

1/4 teaspoon salt substitute

1/4 teaspoon black pepper, freshly ground

tablespoon olive oil

1 tablespoon dried basil, crushed

1 pinch red pepper flakes, crushed

1 pound sea scallops, cut crosswise into halves

1 can (8 ounces) tomato sauce, no-salt-added

1   can (14 1/2 ounces) whole tomatoes, no-salt-added, drain, chop, reserve juice

Directions:

1.   In a large skillet or pan on medium heat. Add the garlic and the shallots; sauté for about 1 minute.

2.   Add the chopped tomatoes with the juice, the tomato sauce, the herbs, and season with the salt and the pepper; stir and simmer for 10 minutes.

3.   Add the scallops; continue cooking gently for 5 minutes, or until the scallops are just cooked through.

4.   Meanwhile, cook the linguine according to the direction of the package until al dente; drain and divide between 4 pasta bowls, about 1 cup for each bowl.

5.   Divide the scallop mixture between the 4 bowls.

6.   If desired, garnish with fresh basil leaves.

7.   Serve with whole-grain Italian bread and tosses green salad.

8. Serve immediately.

Lemon Caper Chicken

Servings: 4

Ingredients

1/2 pounds of Skinless Boneless Chicken Breast Halves (Pounded 3/4 Inch Thick & Cut Into Pieces)

Eggs

Cup of Dry Breadcrumbs

1/2 teaspoon of Ground Black Pepper

tablespoons of Olive Oil

1/4 cup of Capers

Lemons (Cut Into Wedges)

Directions:

1.   Beat your eggs and black pepper together in your bowl. Place your breadcrumbs in a separate bowl.

2.   Heat your olive oil over a medium heat in a large skillet. Dip each piece of your chicken into your egg mixture and press into your breadcrumbs. Brush the loose breadcrumbs off the chicken and place the pieces into your hot oil. Fry in your pan for 5 to 8 minutes per side until golden brown. Remove your chicken from the heat.

3.   Arrange your chicken pieces on a platter, drizzle a small amount of your caper juice over the chicken. Top with the capers and add the lemon wedges.

4.   Serve and Enjoy!

Tuna Sandwiches

Servings: 4

Ingredients:

1/3 cup sun-dried tomato packed in oil, drained 1/4 cup red bell pepper, finely chopped (optional)

1/4 cup red onions or 1/4 cup sweet Spanish onion, finely chopped

1/4 cup ripe green olives or 1/4 cup ripe olives, sliced

1/4 teaspoon black pepper, fresh ground

2   cans (6 ounce) tuna in water, drained, flaked

2 teaspoons capers (more to taste)

4 romaine lettuce or curly green lettuce leaves

4 teaspoons balsamic vinegar

4 teaspoons roasted red pepper

8 slices whole-grain bread (or 8 slices whole-wheat pita bread) Olive oil

Optional:

3 tablespoons mayonnaise (or low-fat mayonnaise)

Directions:

1.   Toast the bread, if desired.

2.   In a small mixing bowl, mix the vinegar and the olive oil. Brush the oil mixture over 1 side of each bread slices or on the inside of the pita pockets.

3.   Except for the lettuce, combine the remaining of the ingredients in a mixing bowl.

4.   Place 1 lettuce leaf on the oiled side of 4 bread slices.

5.   Top the leaves with the tuna mix; top with the remaining bread slices with the oiled side in.

6.   If using pita, place 1 lettuce leave inside each pita slices, then fill with the tuna mixture; serve immediately.

Roasted Summer Vegetables Layers

Servings: 1

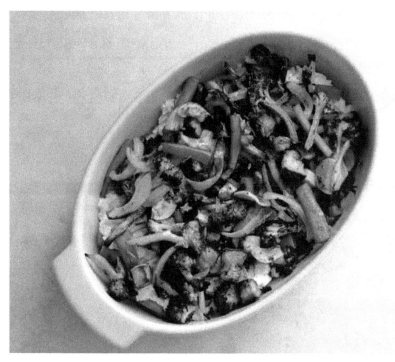

Ingredients:

Large garlic bulb, kept whole

Small bunch rosemary, broken into sprigs
Aubergines/eggplants, sliced

Large courgettes/zucchini, sliced into thick pieces (yellow ones preferred)

Ripe plum tomato, sliced Tablespoons olive oil, good-quality

Directions:

1. Preheat the oven to 220C, gas to 7, or fan to 200C.

2. Grease a round oven-safe dish with a little olive oil

3. Starting from the outside, alternately layer the vegetable slices, making a concentric circle until you fill the dish to the middle. Place the whole garlic in the center of the layer. If there are any leftover vegetable slices, tuck them into gaps in the layer, around the outside. Stick rosemary sprigs between the vegetables and then generously drizzle with olive oil; season with salt and pepper.

4. Roast for about 50 minutes up to 1 hour, or until the layered vegetables are lightly charred and soft.

5. Remove the dish from the dish; let stand for a couple of minutes.

6. Remove the whole garlic head, separate the cloves, and serve for squeezing over the vegetables.

Scallops in a Citrus Sauce

Servings: 4

Ingredients:

2 Teaspoons Olive Oil Shallot, Minced

20 Sea Scallops, Cleaned

1 Teaspoon Lime Zest

1 Tablespoon Lemon Zest Teaspoons Orange Zest

1 Tablespoon Basil, Fresh & Chopped

½ Cup Orange Juice, Fresh Tablespoons Lemon Juice, Fresh 2 Tablespoons Honey, Raw

1 Tablespoon Greek Yogurt, Plain

½ Teaspoon Sea Salt, Fine

Directions:

1.   Get out a large skillet and heat up your olive oil over medium- high heat. Add in your shallot, and sauté for a minute. They should soften.

2.   Add your scallops in, searing for five minutes. Turn once during this time. They should be tender.

3.   Push your scallops to the edge of the skillet, stirring in your three zests, basil, lemon juice and orange juice. Simmer for three minutes.

4.   Whisk in your yogurt, honey and sea salt. Cook for four minutes. Coat your scallops in the sauce before serving warm.

Pork Chops & Wild Mushrooms

Servings: 4

Ingredients:

Tablespoon Olive Oil

4 Pork Chops, Center Cut, Bone In & 5 Ounces Each

 ¼ Teaspoon Sea Salt, Fine

¼ Teaspoon Black Pepper 1 Sweet Onion, Chopped

1 lb. Wild Mushrooms, Sliced Teaspoons Garlic, Minced

1 Teaspoon Thyme, Fresh & Chopped

½ Cup Chicken Stock, Sodium Free

Directions:

1.   Start by patting your pork chops dry using paper towel. Sprinkle your salt and pepper over them, and then get out a large skillet.

2.   Place your skillet over medium-high heat and add in your olive oil. Once your oil is hot, add in your pork chops and cook for another six minutes. Brown them on both sides, and then put them on a plate.

3.   Using the same skillet sauté your garlic and onion for three minutes. They should be fragrant and softened.

4.   Add in your mushrooms and thyme, cooking for six more minutes. Your mushrooms should be tender and lightly caramelized.

5.   Return your pork chops to the skillet and add in your chicken stock. Bring it to a boil while covered, and reduce your heat to low. Allow it to simmer for ten more minutes before serving warm.

Tomato Linguine

Servings: 4

Ingredients:

2 lb. Cherry Tomatoes

2 Tablespoons Balsamic Vinegar

3 Tablespoons Olive Oil

2 Teaspoons Garlic, Minced

¾ lb. Linguine Pasta, Whole Wheat

¼ Teaspoon black Pepper

¼ Cup Feta Cheese, Crumbled Tablespoon Oregano, Fresh & Chopped

Directions:

1.   Start by heating your oven to 350, and then get out a baking sheet. Line your baking sheet with parchment paper before setting it aside.

2.   Get out a bowl and then toss two tablespoons of olive oil, garlic, balsamic vinegar, pepper and tomatoes together until well coated. Spread your tomatoes on your baking sheet, roasting for fifteen minutes. They should soften and burst open.

3.   Cook your pasta according to package directions, and then drain it, placing it in a bowl.

4.   Toss your pasta with the remaining olive oil and add in your tomatoes.

5.   Serve topped with feta and oregano.

Asparagus & Kale Pesto Pasta

Servings: 6

Ingredients:

¼ Cup Basil, Fresh

¾ lb. Asparagus, Trimmed & Chopped Roughly

¼ lb. Kale, Washed

½ Cup Asiago Cheese, Grated

¼ Cup Olive Oil

Lemon, Juiced & Zested

¼ Teaspoon Sea Salt, Fine

¼ Teaspoon Black Pepper 1 lb. Angel Hair Pasta

Directions:

1.   Start by pulsing your kale and asparagus in a food processor until it's finely chopped. Add in your olive oil, lemon juice, basil, and asiago cheese. Continue to pulse until it forms a pesto that's smooth, seasoning with salt and pepper.

2.   Cook your pasta according to package instructions before draining it and placing it in a bowl.

3.   Add in your pesto and make sure to toss to coat. Sprinkle with lemon zest before serving.

Dilly Baked Salmon

Servings: 4

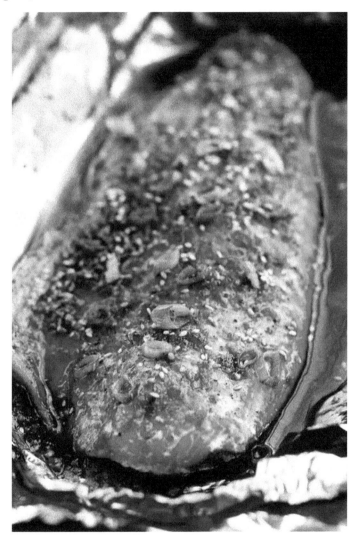

Ingredients

4 (6-ounce) salmon filets

2 tablespoons extra-virgin olive oil

1/2 teaspoon salt

1/4 teaspoon freshly ground black pepper

Juice of large Valencia orange or tangerine

4 teaspoons orange or tangerine zest

4 tablespoons chopped fresh dill

Directions

1.   Preheat the oven to 375°F. Prepare four 10-inch-long pieces of aluminum foil.

2.   Rub each salmon filet on both sides with the olive oil. Season each with salt and pepper and place one in the center of each piece of foil.

3.   Drizzle the orange juice over each piece of fish and top with 1 teaspoon orange zest and 1 tablespoon dill.

4.   For each packet, fold the two long sides of the foil together and then fold the short ends in to make a packet. Make sure to leave about 2 inches of air space within the foil so the fish can steam. Place the packets on a baking sheet.

Mussels with White Wine

Servings: 4

Ingredients

4 pounds fresh, live mussels

2 cups dry white wine 1/2 teaspoon sea salt

6 garlic cloves, minced

4 teaspoons diced shallot

1/2 cup chopped fresh parsley, divided

4 tablespoons extra-virgin olive oil

Juice of 1/2 lemon

Directions

1.   In a large colander, scrub and rinse the mussels under cold water. Discard any mussels that do not close when tapped. Use a paring knife to remove the beard from each mussel.

2.   In a large stock skillet over medium-high heat, bring the wine, salt, garlic, shallots, and 1/4 cup of the parsley to a steady simmer.

3.   Add the mussels, cover, and simmer just until all of the mussels open, 5 to 7 minutes. Do not overcook.

4.   Using a slotted spoon, divide the mussels among 4 large, shallow bowls.

5.   Add the olive oil and lemon juice to the skillet, stir, and pour the broth over the mussels. Garnish each serving with 1

tablespoon of the remaining fresh parsley and serve with a crusty, wholegrain baguette.

Oven-Poached Cod

Servings: 4

Ingredients

4 (6-ounce) cod filets 1/2 teaspoon salt

1/2 teaspoon freshly ground black pepper

1/2 cup dry white wine

1/2 cup seafood or vegetable stock 2 garlic cloves, minced

1 bay leaf

1 teaspoon chopped fresh sage 4 rosemary sprigs for garnish

Directions

1.   Preheat the oven to 375°F.

2.   Season each filet with salt and pepper and place in a large ovenproof skillet or baking pan. Add the wine, stock, garlic, bay leaf, and sage and cover. Bake until the fish flakes easily with a fork, about 20 minutes.

3.   Use a spatula to remove the filet from the skillet. Place the poaching liquid over high heat and cook, stirring frequently, until reduced by half, about 10 minutes. (Do this in a small saucepan if you used a baking pan.)

4.   To serve, place a filet on each plate and drizzle with the reduced poaching liquid. Garnish each with a fresh rosemary sprig.

Flank Steak Spinach Salad

Servings: 4

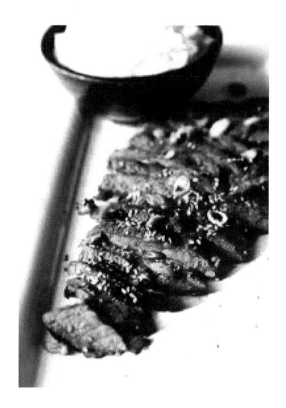

Ingredients

1 pound flank steak

1 teaspoon extra-virgin olive oil 1 tablespoon garlic powder

1/2 teaspoon salt

1/2 teaspoon freshly ground black pepper

4 cups baby spinach leaves 10 cherry tomatoes, halved

10 cremini or white mushrooms, sliced

1 small red onion, thinly sliced 1/2 red bell pepper, thinly sliced

Directions

1.   Preheat the broiler. Line a baking sheet with aluminum foil.

2.   Rub the top of the flank steak with the olive oil, garlic powder, salt, and pepper and let sit for 10 minutes before placing under the broiler. Broil for 5 minutes on each side for medium rare. Allow the meat to rest on a cutting board for 10 minutes.

3.   Meanwhile, in a large bowl, combine the spinach, tomatoes, mushrooms, onion, and bell pepper and toss well.

4.   To serve, divide the salad among 4 dinner plates. Slice the steak on the diagonal and place 4 to 5 slices on top of each salad. Serve with your favorite vinaigrette.

Hearty Chicken and Vegetable Soup

Servings: 2

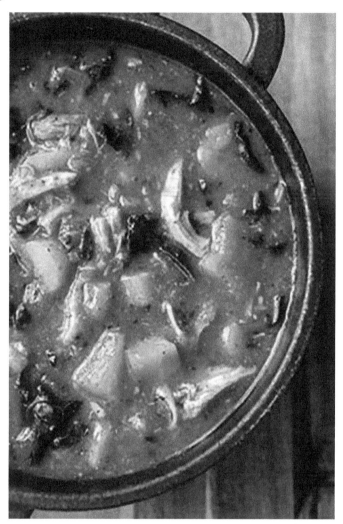

Ingredients

1   teaspoon extra-virgin olive oil 1 medium yellow onion, diced 1 large carrot, peeled and diced 1 celery stalk, peeled and diced

2   (6-ounce) boneless, skinless chicken breasts, cut into 1-inch pieces

1 medium zucchini, diced 2 yellow squash, diced

1/2 cup chopped fresh parsley, plus extra for garnish 1 teaspoon chopped fresh oregano

1 teaspoon chopped fresh basil 1/2 teaspoon salt

1/4 teaspoon freshly ground black pepper 2 cups chicken stock

Directions

1.   In a large, heavy skillet, heat the olive oil over medium-high heat. Add the onion, carrot, and celery and sauté, stirring frequently, for 5 minutes. Add the chicken and continue to sauté

for another 10 minutes, stirring often.

2.   Add the zucchini and squash, then the parsley, oregano, basil, salt, and pepper. Sauté for 5 minutes, reduce the heat to medium, and pour in the stock. Cover and cook for an additional 10 minutes.

3.   To serve, ladle into bowls and garnish with additional parsley.

Fettuccine with Tomatoes and Pesto

Servings: 4

Ingredients

1 pound whole-grain fettuccine

4 Roma tomatoes, diced 2 teaspoons tomato paste 1 cup vegetable broth

2 garlic cloves, minced

1 tablespoon chopped fresh oregano

1/2 teaspoon salt

1 packed cup fresh basil leaves 1/4 cup extra-virgin olive oil 1/4 cup grated Parmesan cheese

1/4 cup pine nuts

Directions

1.   Bring a large stock skillet of water to a boil over high heat and cook the fettuccine according to the package instructions until al dente (still slightly firm). Drain but do not rinse.

2.   Meanwhile, in a large, heavy skillet, combine the tomatoes, tomato paste, broth, garlic, oregano, and salt and stir well. Cook over medium heat for 10 minutes.

3.   In a blender or food processor, combine the basil, olive oil, Parmesan cheese, and pine nuts and blend until smooth.

4.   Serve immediately.

Dirty Potatoes

Servings: 3

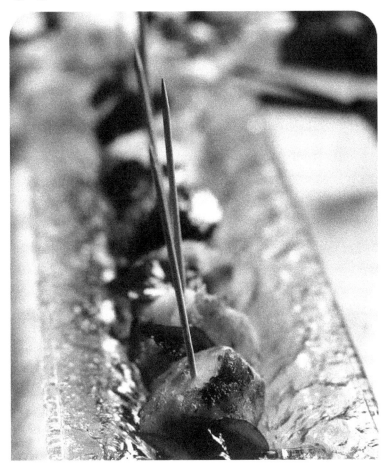

Ingredients

- 2 lbs. small potatoes
- 2 tbsps. olive oil
- 0.33 c. pitted kalamata olives

Directions:

1. Bake the potatoes for 400 F until it's cooked.

2.   Use food processor for the olives, and serve it together with the cooked potatoes.

Chicken Cordon Bleu Recipe

Servings: 4

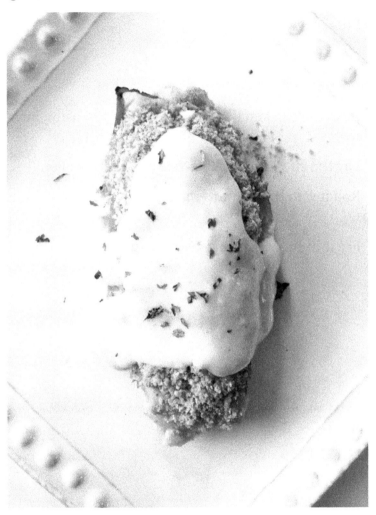

Ingredients

- 2 pcs. chicken breast fillet
- 2 slices ham
- 4 slices cheddar cheese
- 2 oz. bread crumbs

- Season flour to coat

- 1 large egg

- Milk of choice

- Salt and black pepper

Directions:

1. Bash the chicken fillet as thin as you can using meat hammer.

2. Lay the cheese on the hammered chicken fillet.

3. Roll it into the flour, to the egg, and lastly in bread crumbs.

4. Fry it in the pan using olive oil until golden brown.

Prawns in Garlic

Servings: 3

Ingredients

- 2 lbs. shrimps

- 4 cloves garlic-finely chopped
- 2 dried red chilies
- 1 large lemon
- 1 bunch parsley-chopped
- 1 c olive oil

- Salt
- Spanish bread

Directions:

1. Mix all the ingredients and oven the shrimp for 200c , after cooking serve it with bread.

Sword Fish Steaks

Servings: 6

Ingredients

- 6 pcs. Sword fish steaks – 8 oz. each

- 2 tbsps. olive oil

- Salt and black pepper

- 1 pack tomato salsa

Directions:

1. Marinate the fish steaks with olive oil, salt, and black pepper.

2. Preheat the pack of tomato salsa.

3. Fry the steaks in olive oil until golden brown and serve with tomato salsa.

Grilled Fish

Servings: 4

Ingredients

- 450 g rosada fillet
- 1 c olive oil
- Salt and black pepper
- 2 cloves garlic-finely chopped
- 1 c lemon juice
- Handful of chopped parsley

Directions:

1. Marinate the rosada with salt and black pepper with olive oil for an hour.

2. Cook the marinated rosada in a pan until golden brown.

3. Mix the garlic, lemon juice, and parsley to make the sauce, pour it to the cooked rosada, and serve.

Garlic Linguine

Servings: 4

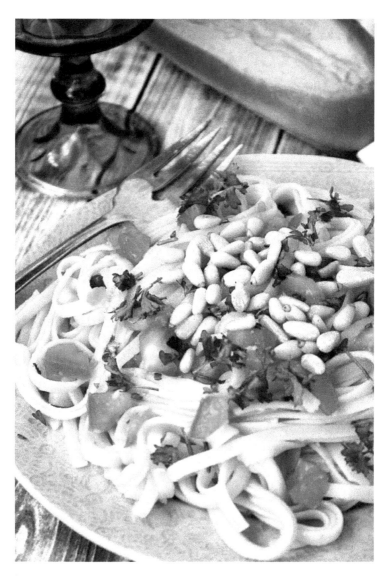

Ingredients

- 1 pack linguini pasta
- 2 tbsps. olive oil

- 1 tbsp. minced garlic
- 1 tbsp. dried basil
- 1 tbsp. dried oregano
- 1 tsp. dried thyme
- 2 c chopped tomatoes

Directions:

1. Prepare and cook pasta as per pack suggestions.
2. Cook the garlic and herbs in olive oil for 2 minutes.
3. Put the linguini and fold in the tomatoes and serve.

Simple Lemon Herb Chicken

Servings: 2

Ingredients

- 2 chicken breasts

- 2 sprigs fresh parsley

- 1 lemon

- Salt and pepper

- 1 tbsp. olive oil

- 1 pinch dried oregano

Directions:

1. Squeeze lemon on chicken, add salt and pepper, and cook in olive oil.

2. Add the remaining ingredients and serve.

Broiled Herb Buttered Chicken

Servings: 4

Ingredients

- 4 pcs. Chicken breast
- ½ c butter-softened
- 3 cloves garlic-minced
- 1 tsp. dried parsley
- ¼ tsp. dried rosemary
- ¼ tsp. dried thyme

Directions:

1. Combine garlic, butter, parsley, rosemary, and thyme, and spread evenly on each chicken breast.

2. Grill in the oven until golden brown or 15 minutes and serve.

Lemon Marinated Chicken

Servings: 8

Ingredients

- ½ c lemon juice
- 2 tbsps. vinegar
- 3 tbsps. dried oregano
- 1 tsp. paprika
- ¼ tsp. black pepper
- ½ onion-chopped
- ½ lemon zest
- 4 pcs. skinless chicken breast

Directions:

1. Mix the vinegar, oregano, paprika, lemon juice. onion, and

lemon zest, and let it stand for 4 hours.

2. Bake the chicken for 30 minutes, and serve.

Terry's Lemon Caper Chicken

Servings: 4

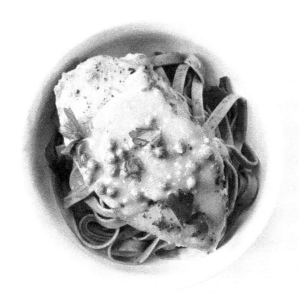

Ingredients

- 2 pcs. eggs
- ½ tbsp. black pepper
- 1 cup breadcrumbs
- 2 tbsps. olive oil

- 1 ½ boneless chicken beast
- ¼ c capers
- 2 lemons-wedge cuts

Directions:

1. Beat eggs with black pepper, prepare the breadcrumbs, and set aside.

2. Fry the chicken, dip first in the egg, then put in the breadcrumbs and cook for 8 minutes.

3. Serve with capers and lemon wedges.

Maple-chili Glazed Pork

Servings: 6

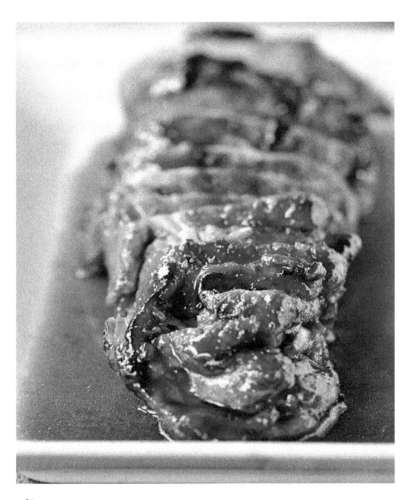

Ingredients

- 1 tsp. chili powder

- ½ tsp. salt

- 1/8 tsp. ground Chipotle pepper

- 1 pound pork tenderloin

- 2 tsps. Canada oil

- ¼ c apple cider

- 1 tbsp. maple syrup

- 1 tsp. cider vinegar

Directions:

1.   Combine salt, ground Chipotle, and chili powder. Rub on each sides of the pork.

2.   Fry the pork with oil until golden, add vinegar, syrup, and cider to the pan, cook for 3 minutes, and serve.

Barbecued Chicken Burritos

Servings: 2

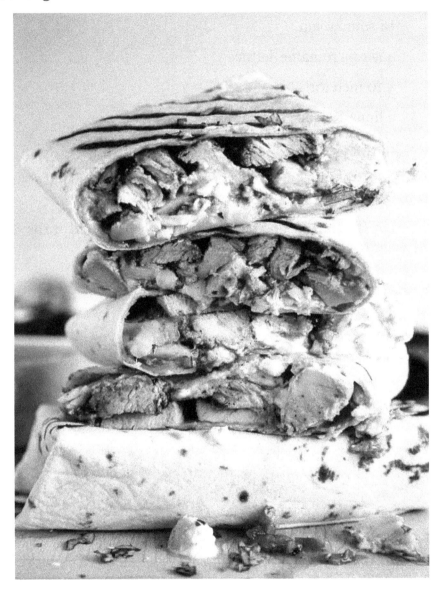

Ingredients

- 1 2 pound roasted chicken
- ½ c barbecue sauce

- 1 c black beans
- ½ c canned corn
- ¼ sour cream
- 4 leaves romaine-lettuce
- 4 10 inch tortillas
- 2 limes-wedge cut

Directions:

1.   Cook the chicken, beans, barbecue sauce, corn, and sour cream for 5 minutes.

2.   Lay the tortilla, and top it with the chicken mixture as well as lettuce, and serve.

Chicken and Fruit Salad

Servings: 4

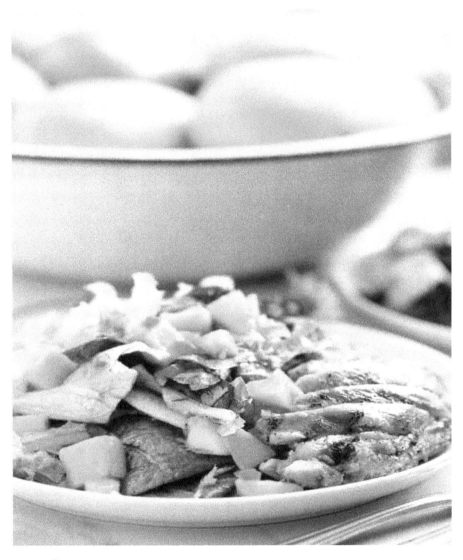

Ingredients

- ¼ c sour cream

- 3 tbsps. fruit flavored vinegar

- 4 tsps. sugar

- 1 ½ tsp. poppy seeds
- ¼ tsp. salt
- Pepper

- 8 c mixed salad greens
- 2 cups sliced cooked chicken breast
- 2 c melon-chopped
- ¼ c toasted walnut
- ¼ crumbled feta cheese

Directions:

1. Mix all the ingredients, arrange it in choice, and serve.

Broccoli with Feta Omelet and Toast

Servings: 4

Ingredients

- Cooking spray
- 1 c chopped broccoli
- 2 large eggs-beaten
- 2 tbsps. feta cheese
- ¼ teaspoon dried dill
- 2 toasted bread

Directions:

2. Coat pan with a cooking spray, add broccoli- cook for 3 minutes.

3. Mix feta, eggs and dill. Add it to the pan and let it cook; turn the omelet to cook for other side and serve.

Banana Almond toast

Servings: 4

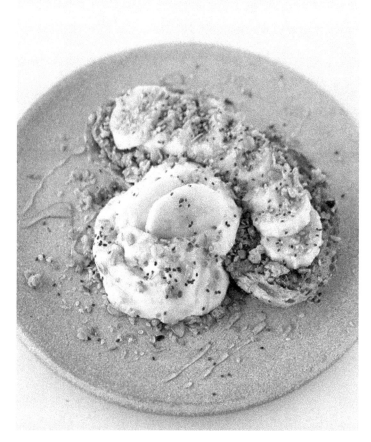

Ingredients

- 1 tbsp. almond butter
- 1 slice rye bread-toasted
- 1 banana-sliced

Directions:

1. Spread the almond butter on the toast, top it with banana, and serve.

BBQ Turkey Burger

Servings: 4

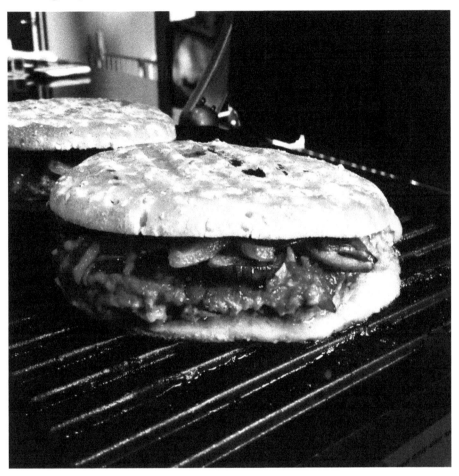

Ingredients

- 1 pound turkey meat
- 1 garlic clove-minced
- ½ tsp. paprika

- ¼ tsp. cumin

- Salt

- ½ tsp. black pepper

- 4 slices grilled-onions

- ¼ c bbq sauce

- 4 sesame seed buns-toasted

Directions:

1. Make the patty by mixing turkey meat, garlic, cumin, and paprika.

2. Fry this patty seasoned with salt and pepper and serve it as burger.

Middle Eastern Rice Salad

Servings: 5

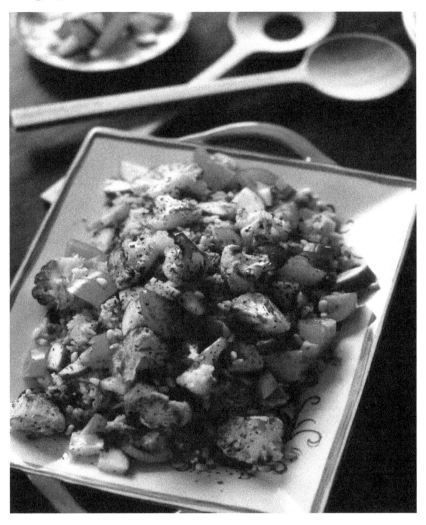

Ingredients

- 2 tbsps. olive oil
- ½ Vidalia

- 1 can chickpeas
- ½ tbsp. cumin
- ¼ salt
- Black pepper
- 3 cups cooked brown rice
- ½ c chopped pitted dates
- ¼ c mint-chopped
- ¼ c parsley-chopped

Directions:

1.	Cook the onions first, and add the chickpeas, cumin, and salt and pepper.

2.	Add the rice, dates, parsley, and mint, and serve.

Pan Grilled Salmon with Pineapple Salsa

Servings: 4

Ingredients

- 1 cup pineapple-chopped
- 2 tbsps. chopped onion
- 2 tbsps. chopped cilantro
- 1 tbsp. rice vinegar
- 1/ 8 tsp. red pepper
- 4 salmon fillets
- ½ tsp. Salt

Directions:

1. Mix the firsts 5 ingredients.
2. Cook the salmon, top with the salsa, and serve.

Italian Garbanzo Salad

Servings: 4

Ingredients

- 3 cup fennel bulb-chopped

- 2 cup tomato-chopped
- 1 ¾ c onion-chopped
- 1 cup basil-chopped
- 1/3 cup balsamic vinegar
- 1 tbsp. olive oil
- 1 tsp. black pepper
- ¼ tsp. salt
- 4 cloves garlic-minced
- 2 cans chickpeas
- ½ c crumbled feta cheese

Directions:

1. Mix all the ingredients, sprinkle the top with cheese, and serve

White Bean and Herb Hummus

Servings: 2

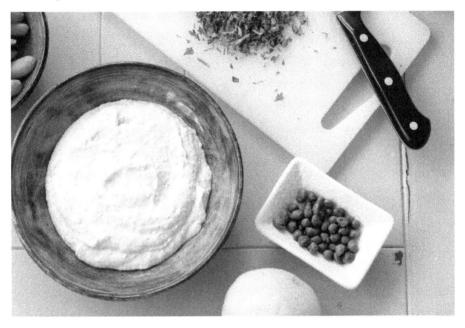

Ingredients

- ¼ cup canned white beans-drained

- 1 tbsp. chopped chives

- 1 tbsp. lemon juice

- 2 tsps. olive oil

- Assorted raw vegetables of choice

Directions:

1.   Combine all ingredients, mash it, and serve with vegetables of choice.

Greek Salad with Sardines

Servings: 3

Ingredients

- 3 tbsps. lemon juice
- 2 tbsps. olive oil
- 1 clove garlic-minced

- 2 tsps. dried oregano
- ½ tsp. ground pepper
- 3 tomatoes-chunks cut
- 1 cucumber-chunks cut
- 1 15 ounce can chickpeas
- 1/3 c crumbled feta cheese
- ¼ c onion
- 2 tbsps. kalamata olives
- A can of sardines

Directions:

1. Combine all ingredients, and top it with sardines.

Artichoke and Ripe-Olive Tuna Salad

Servings: 6

Ingredients

- 1 12 ounce can chunk light tuna-flaked
- 1 c artichoke-chopped
- ½ c olives-chopped
- 1/3 c mayonnaise
- 2 tsps. lemon juice
- 1 ½ oregano-chopped

Directions:

1. Mix artichokes, mayonnaise, tuna, olives, lemon juice, and oregano in a bowl and serve.

Easy lemon and Herb Blackened Chicken

Servings: 2

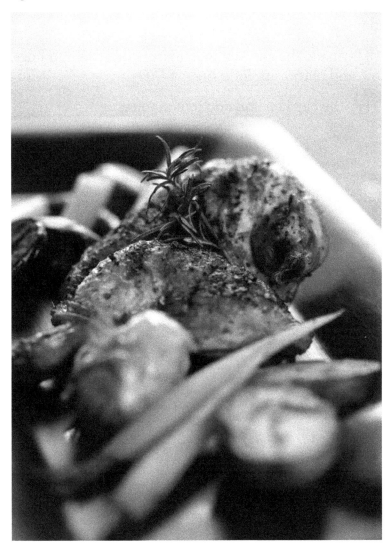

Ingredients

- 1 c lemon juice

- 2 tbsps. olive oil

- 2 tbsps. dried marjoram

- 4 pcs. Boneless chicken breast

- 1 tbsp. lemon juice

Directions:

1. Marinade the chicken in a mixture of 1 c lemon juice, olive oil, and marjoram for 2 hrs.

2. Fry the chicken and add lemon juice.

Lemon Pepper Chicken

Servings: 6

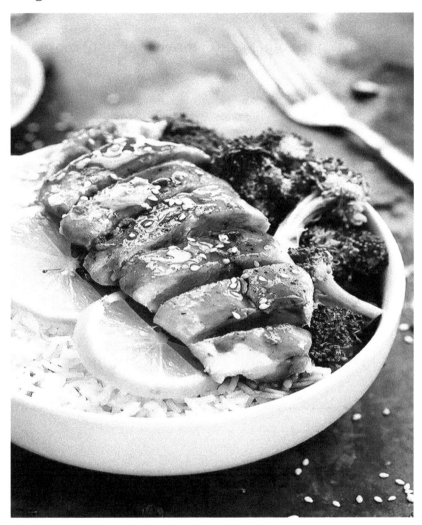

Ingredients

- 2 tsps. butter

- 1 tbsp. black pepper

- 1 skinless boneless chicken breast

- 1 tbsp. lemon juice

Directions:

1.   Cook chicken in a pan, add pepper, lemon juice for 7 minutes.

2.   Do this on the other side of the chicken until cooked, and serve.

Penne with Garlic Pesto

Servings: 4

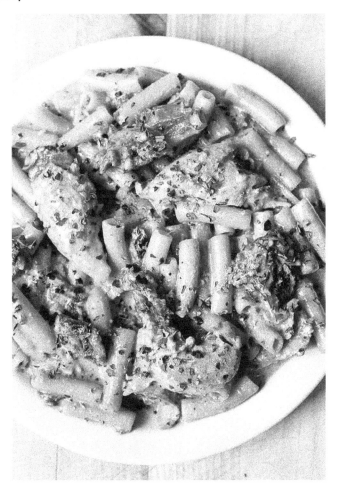

Ingredients

- 2/3 c vegetable stock

- 2 cloves garlic

- 1 c packed basil leaves

- 1/3 c grated Parmesan Cheese

- 2 tbsps. pine nuts

- 12 ounces penne pasta

- 2 large tomatoes-chopped

Directions:

1. Cook pasta first, add salt.

2. Cook stock and garlic cloves, for 5 minutes.

3. Use food processor for basil, add stock mixture , parmesan cheese, and nuts, and pour into the pasta and serve.

Grilled Shrimps

Servings: 5

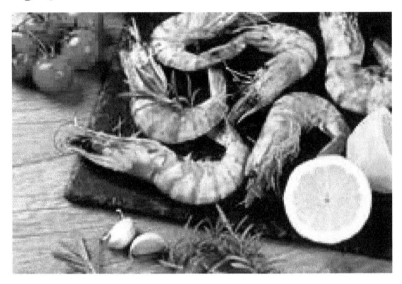

Ingredients

- 800 unshelled large prawns
- 2 cloves garlic-crushed
- 3 dried chilies
- 1 c lime zest
- 1 c coriander-chopped
- 4 tbsps. olive oil
- Salt and black pepper

Directions:

1. Marinate the shrimp with garlic, chilies, lime zest, coriander, olive oil, salt, and pepper.

2. Use wooden skewers, and enjoy grilling.

Chicken and Mushroom with Fresh Asparagus

Servings: 6

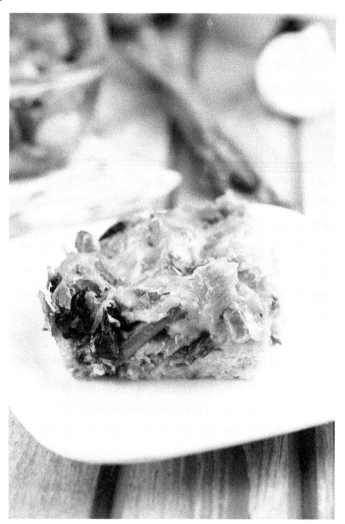

Ingredients

- 4 pcs. chicken meat

- 12 mushrooms

- 24 asparagus tips

- 2 cloves garlic-finely chopped

- 3 tbsps. cognac to flambé

- 1 large glass of cherry

- Olive oil

- Salt and black pepper

Directions:

1.   Fry the chicken meat in olive oil until skin gets crispy and cooked.

2.   Fry the mushrooms and asparagus, then garlic.

3.   Assemble the cooked ingredients and serve.

Smoked Mackerel Sandwich

Servings: 4

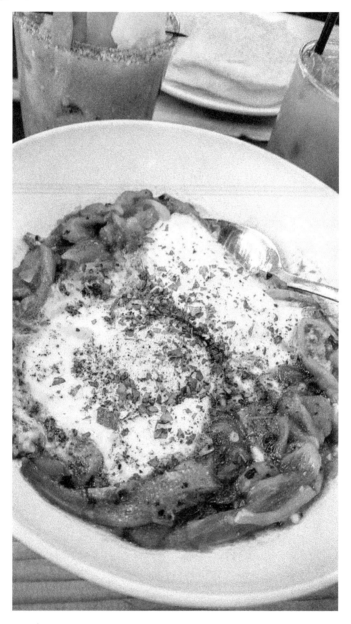

Ingredients

- 1 large garlic

- 1 tsp. olive oil

- 9 slices of Italian bread

- Salt

- Small arugula leaves

- 3 smoked mackerel fillets

- ½ tbsp. onion

- 2 medium size tomatoes

Directions:

1. Bake the garlic for 350 F for 40 minutes and set aside.

2. Grill the bread brushed with olive oil.

3. Extract the roasted garlic in a bowl with salt, olive oil.

4. Lay the grilled bread and top with the garlic mixture, mackerel, onion, and tomato slices.

Hasselback Caprese Chicken

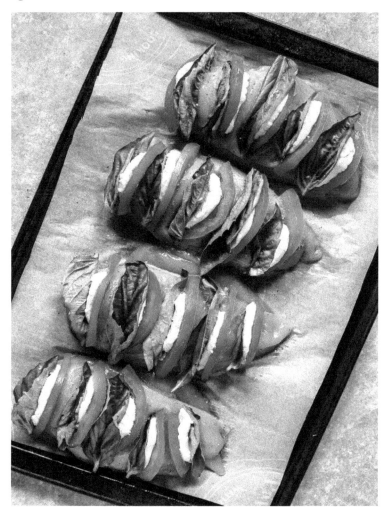

Ingredients

- 1/2 tsp. salt, divided

- 3 oz. fresh mozzarella, halved and sliced
- 2 chicken breasts, boneless and skinless

- 1/2 tsp. black pepper, divided
- 1 medium tomato, sliced
- 1/4 cup prepared pesto
- 2 tbsp. extra virgin olive oil
- 8 cups broccoli florets

Directions

1. Preheat the oven to 370 degrees F and grease a baking sheet.

2. Season the chicken with salt and black pepper.

3. Insert mozzarella and tomato slices in the chicken cuts.

4. Brush with pesto and transfer the chicken breasts on the baking sheet.

5. Toss broccoli with oil, salt and black pepper in a large bowl.

6. Spread the broccoli mixture around the chicken and bake for about 25 minutes.

7. Dish out and serve warm. Enjoy!

Olive Chicken

Servings: 6

Ingredients

- 2 tbsp. white wine
- 3 garlic cloves, minced
- 2 tsp. olive oil
- 6 chicken breast halves, skinless and boneless
- 1/2 cup onions, diced
- 1/2 cup white wine
- 1 tbsp. fresh basil, chopped
- 2 fennel bulbs, sliced in half
- Salt and black pepper, to taste
- 3 cups tomatoes, chopped
- 2 tsp. fresh thyme, chopped
- 1/2 cup kalamata olives
- 1/4 cup fresh parsley, chopped

Directions

1. Heat oil with 2 tablespoons white wine in a large skillet on medium heat.

2. Add chicken and cook for about 6 minutes per side.

3. Transfer the chicken to a plate and stir in garlic.

4. Sauté for about 30 seconds and add onions.

5. Sauté for about 3 minutes and stir in fennel and tomatoes.

6. Allow it to boil and lower the heat.

7. Add half cup white wine and cook for about 10 minutes.

8. Stir in basil and thyme and cook for about 5 minutes.

9. Return the cooked chicken to the skillet.

10. Cover the cooking pan and cook on low heat.

11. Stir in parsley and olives and cook for about 1 minute.

12. Adjust seasoning with salt and black pepper. Serve and enjoy!

Chicken Souvlaki with Tzatziki Sauce

Servings: 1

Ingredients

- 1/4 cup virgin olive oil
- 3 tbsp. fresh lemon juice
- 2 garlic cloves, minced
- 2 tsp. chopped fresh oregano
- 3/4 tsp. kosher salt, to taste
- 1/4 tsp. freshly ground black pepper
- 4 tbsp. red wine vinegar
- 4 boneless, skinless chicken breasts, cut into 1 1/2 inch wide strips
- For the Tzatziki Sauce:
- 1 medium cucumber, peeled and sliced
- Kosher salt, to taste
- Freshly ground black pepper
- 2 garlic cloves, minced
- 1/3 cup chopped dill, fresh
- 2 cups plain fat-free Greek yogurt

- 1 1/2 tbsp. fresh lemon juice

Directions

1. In a large bowl, whisk together, oil, juice, garlic, oregano, salt, pepper and vinegar. Add chicken, tossing to coat in marinade.

2. Cover and refrigerate 30 minutes or up to 1 hour.

3. Meanwhile, soak wooden skewers in cold water.

4. For the Tzatziki Sauce: Add cucumbers to a colander and sprinkle generously with salt. Let cucumbers drain for 30 minutes, tossing occasionally.

5. Add cucumber, garlic, dill, yogurt and lemon juice to a blender. Season with pepper. Blend until smooth and creamy.

6. Transfer to a bowl, cover and refrigerate.

7. Preheat oven to 425°F.

8. Remove chicken from marinade and thread onto skewers. Discard marinade.

9. Arrange skewers on a foil-lined baking sheet with a rack.

10. Bake 7 to 9 minutes, turning once, or until chicken is no longer pink in the middle. Transfer to serving plates.

11. Serve with tzatziki sauce on the side for dipping. Enjoy!

Weeknight Tandoori Chicken

Servings: 4

Ingredients

- 2 cups Greek yogurt
- 4 tsp. minced garlic
- 4 tsp. paprika
- 4 tsp. ground coriander
- 2 tsp. ground cumin
- 2 tsp. minced ginger
- 1 tsp. red pepper flakes
- Juice of 1 lime
- Kosher salt, to taste
- Freshly ground black pepper
- 1 1/2 lb. boneless, skinless chicken thighs
- Chopped fresh cilantro

Directions

1. In a large bowl, combine yogurt, garlic, paprika, coriander, cumin, ginger, red pepper flakes and half the lime juice. Dredge chicken in yogurt mixture.

2. Cover and let stand 30 minutes.

3. Preheat broiler.

4. Line a rimmed baking sheet with aluminum foil. Transfer chicken breast to pan, bottom side up. Reserve marinade.

5. Broil 3 to 4 minutes or until lightly browned.

6.   Turn chicken over and pour remaining marinade over the top.

7.   Broil 3 to 4 minutes or until lightly browned on the top.

8.   Drizzle remaining lime juice over chicken. Transfer to serving plates.

9.   Spoon some of the cooked yogurt mixture over the chicken. Garnish with cilantro.

10.   Serve remaining yogurt mixture on the side.

Enjoy!

11.   Optionally, you can serve with a side of basmati rice and drizzle the remaining yogurt mixture over the top. You can also serve with sautéed spinach on the side.

Mediterranean Stuffed Chicken

Servings: 3

Ingredients

- 1/3 cup crumbled feta cheese
- 3 sun dried tomatoes (in oil), drained and diced
- 3 tbsp. finely chopped walnuts
- 4 black olives (preferably kalamata), chopped
- 1 lemon, zest and juice
- 2 tsp. ground oregano
- 2 boneless, skinless chicken breasts, about 5 oz. each
- 8 freshly basil leaves
- 1 tsp. extra virgin olive oil
- Kosher salt and freshly ground black pepper, to taste

Directions

1. Preheat oven to 400°F.

2. In a small bowl, combine the feta cheese, tomatoes, walnuts, olives, 2 tsp. lemon zest, 2 tsp. lemon juice and oregano. Set aside.

3. Place chicken breasts between 2 sheets of plastic wrap. Using a mallet, pound chicken to 1/2 inch thick.

4. Place 3 to 4 basil leaves on each breast, leaving 1/2-inch space from edges.

5. Spoon half of cheese mixture in the center of each breast.

6. Starting with the narrower end, roll up the breast up tightly. Use 2 to 3 toothpicks to secure rolls. Brush rollups with oil.

7. Season with salt and pepper

8. Bake for 25 minutes or until an instant-read thermometer inserted into the thickest part registers 165°F and chicken is no longer pink inside. Serve and enjoy!

9. Note that the chicken rollups can be prepared ahead of time. Store in an airtight container in the refrigerator up to 2 days. Add 5 to 10 minutes to cooking time.

Braised Chicken Breasts with Bulgur Pilaf

Servings: 4

Ingredients

- 4 boneless, skinless chicken breasts, about 5 oz. each
- Kosher salt and freshly ground black pepper
- 1/3 cup virgin olive oil
- 1 cup fine-grind bulgur
- 10 oz. cherry tomatoes, halved
- 1/2 cup pitted kalamata, olives, halved
- 4 oz. feta cheese, crumbled
- 3/4 cup minced fresh parsley

- 1 tbsp. fresh lemon juice

Directions

1. Season chicken with salt and pepper.

2. In a large skillet over medium-high heat, add 1 tbsp. oil and heat until shimmering.

3. Cook breasts, turning once, 8 minutes or until browned and no longer pink in the middle.

4. Transfer chicken to cutting board and tent with foil.

5. Add 1-1/2 cups water to the skillet and cook, scraping up any browned bits from the bottom of the pan, until mixture begins to boil. Stir in 2 tsp. salt and bulgur. Remove from the heat.

6.   Cover and let stand 5 minutes, or until bulgur is al dente.

7.   Fluff bulgur with a fork. Stir in tomatoes, olives, feta, parsley, lemon juice and 2 tbsp. oil.

8.   Season to taste with salt and pepper.

9.   Slice chicken across the grain. Spoon bulgur onto serving plates.

10.   Arrange chicken on and around bulgur.

11.   Serve drizzled with remaining oil. Enjoy!

Moroccan Chicken with Oranges and Olives

Servings: 4

Ingredients

- ½ cup rice flour
- 1 teaspoon ground cumin
- 1 teaspoon ground ginger
- 1 teaspoon ground cinnamon
- ½ teaspoon salt
- ¼ teaspoon freshly ground black pepper
- 4 boneless, skinless chicken breasts
- 3 tablespoons extra-virgin olive oil
- 1 garlic clove, thinly sliced
- ½ cup wine
- ½ cup chicken broth or water

- Several saffron threads
- ½ cup salt-cured olives
- 1 orange, sliced
- ¼ cup chopped fresh cilantro

Directions

1.   Combine the rice flour, cumin, ginger, cinnamon, salt, and pepper in a small shallow bowl.

2.   Dredge each piece of chicken in the spice mixture.

3.   Place a large skillet over high heat and add the olive oil. Add the chicken and brown on all sides, about 3 to 4 minutes per side.

4.   Add the garlic, wine, broth or water, and saffron to the pan and bring to a boil. Reduce to a simmer and cook for 15 minutes.

5.   Add the olives and orange slices, cover, and turn off the heat. Let it sit for 5 minutes to combine the flavors.

6.   Remove the lid, add the cilantro, and serve.

7.   This dish can be stored for 5 days in the refrigerator.

Spanish Almond Chicken

Servings: 4

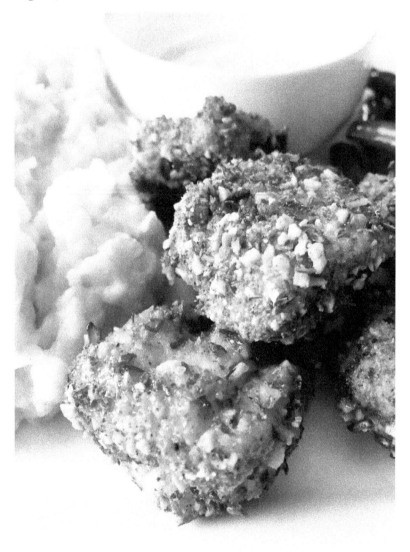

Ingredients

- 1 tablespoon extra-virgin olive oil

- 1 tablespoon butter

- 4 boneless, skinless chicken breasts
- ½ medium onion, sliced
- 1 garlic clove, sliced
- ¼ cup blanched (skinless) unsalted almonds
- ½ teaspoon ground cinnamon
- ½ teaspoon ground nutmeg
- ¼ teaspoon ground turmeric
- ½ cup chicken broth
- ¼ cup dry sherry
- 1 teaspoon salt
- ¼ teaspoon freshly ground black pepper
- 1 tablespoon chopped fresh flatleaf parsley

Directions

1. Place a large skillet over high heat. Add the olive oil and butter and cook the chicken breasts on all sides until firm, about 5 to 7 minutes per side. Remove the chicken and set aside.

2. Add the onion, garlic, almonds, cinnamon, nutmeg, and turmeric to the same pan and sauté until the almonds are lightly browned, about 1 to 2 minutes.

3. Place the almond mixture, chicken broth, sherry, salt, and pepper in a blender or food processor and process until the mixture is smooth. If the sauce is too thick, add additional chicken broth to get the consistency of heavy cream.

4. Return the chicken to the pan and add the almond sauce. Reduce the heat to low and let the sauce warm through. Be careful not to simmer the sauce, because it will separate.

5.   Arrange the chicken and sauce on a serving platter, top with parsley, and serve.

6.   This recipe can be stored in the refrigerator for 4 days.